Another Level

Kinetics

Presents the Fundamentals of Training

By: Leonard Smith

ISBN: 978-1-950088-06-5

Dedication

To my lefty and my righty

Arianna & Khanh Nam

I'll love you until infinity.

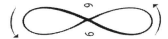

Acknowledgment

I would like to thank all my friends who encouraged me to grow in my career as a fitness trainer. Also, I would express my appreciation for my early clients; working with them helped me to recognize my passion for training and proved to be the impetus that I needed to become certified. I would not be here if I were not surrounded by a supportive circle, which continues to cheer me on as I reach the various milestones of my life.

About The Author

Leonard Smith was born in Gainesville, Florida, but currently calls New York City his home. He has lived in NYC for four years now. His drive to transform lives through fitness training brought and kept him in the city. He has transformed many athletes over the years by being their fitness coach.

He began his unofficial career by working out with people around his neighborhood. Word got out, and more people approached him to help them get fit. Leonard began to train college students at the local apartment complex. Then, he got certified. Since then, there has been no stopping him. His passion for fitness began as a part-time job and changed into a fulltime one. He has developed his craft over the years and has written this book to help people become fit through the right training regimen.

An athletic person, Leonard has won numerous trophies from the different sports he has played throughout his life. He loves basketball and football. He has also wrestled, skate boarded, freestyled on bikes, written poetry, and dabbled in music. He runs six miles a day, likes getting tattoos and has many friends, though he says he needs his alone time to recharge.

Preface

You train, and you train, and you train – but your body does not reflect your hard work. Or, you don't train and want to, but you just don't know how to get started.In both cases, you need instructions to get over that invisible hurdle that stops you from achieving your fitness goals. You have come to the right place: this book is for you. Leonard Smith, longtime fitness trainer, knows the fitness needs and quirks of the human body.

He says, *"It won't cut it to only train; you have to train right!"* Many people input a lot of effort but get little to no rewards from their training. It's because they don't know what they are doing wrong, and what they need to do correctly, to become fit, remain fit and keep getting fitter. In *Another Level Kinetics,* Smith has provided a short and crisp guideline on physical training.

You don't need to stumble about on google for your fitness problems anymore. This short manual on training will help you discover all that you need to insert, delete and modify in your fitness plan. Learn your body, identify its requirements, and structure your exercise regimen to suit it. Remember to keep training right. That's the only way to get to your fitness goal!

Contents

Page Left Blank Intentionally

Chapter 1 – The Start

At *Another Level Kinetics*, we provide fitness and wellbeing for people. Your fitness status does not matter: you may be a beginner, at the intermediate level or an advanced fitness guru. *Another Level Kinetics* caters to the needs of people at every stage of fitness. Every life we touch becomes part of our community, from the mundane to the high arcane.

Here, I, Leonard Smith, owner of *Another Levels Kinetics*, will present ten key points for those who want to start exercising and live a healthy life. In my eleven years as a personal trainer, I have gathered information about training. I have compiled the gist of training tips and lessons in this book. My intent is to help everybody who has an interest in fitness.

So let's begin.

Physical Exam

First things first. If you haven't exercised in a while, or if you have and you are now trying to take it on to the next level you should get a physical done. This is one of the most important steps in creating a healthier you. Most people say,

"It's not really that serious, I'm just going to exercise a little."
Well, if you knew the changes your body goes through when you exercise, you would understand that it is that serious. Imagine you start exercising three days a week. You do this for a year straight. Now, that is a lot of training, everything combined. However, you find that your body still does not produce the results that you want; it might also not produce any results at all.

That is like working at a job for a year straight but never getting paid. This is what happens to a lot of people who train. And I can tell you that it can be extremely frustrating. This is exactly the kind of frustration that might make you want to give up. For example, I knew a girl named Racheal. She was 30 years old when she did personal training with a trainer at a certain gym I use to work at. I would see Racheal come into the gym at least three times a week: on Monday, Wednesday and Friday.

I knew this because she always trained at 7 pm the exact days and time that I would train one of my clients named Maria. Now, Rachel and Maria would see each other so much that it soon started to become a competition of who trained the hardest during their training session. Whatever one did the other would try to outdo her if some of the same exercises were in the other's program for that day. Over a period of two to three months, Maria, my client, lost at least 15 Lbs.

Her body just went to take on a shape and form of its own. Every time I turned around people were complimenting her progress. Her results were starting to show more and more each day. I should mention that Maria had a positive outlook and a healthy attitude toward life. Her energy was vibrant. As time went by, Maria and Rachel became friends and started to hang outside of the gym.

Their conversation did not only focus on the topic of training. They would talk about what types of food they liked to eat, and what time the other made it in last night from partying. Pretty soon, Rachel began to get a little concerned. She started wondering, *"Why am I not seeing any results at all?"*

I remember it like it was yesterday. Maria asked me before one of our training sessions, *"Will you train Rachel?"*

I said, *"Why are you asking me that question? Isn't she still training with Johnny?"* Johnny was one of the trainers of the club at that time and was a friend of mine.

Maria said, *"Yes, but Racheal thinks Johnny doesn't know what he's doing because her body hasn't changed at all in six months. She's starting to get worried."*

I told Maria, *"Well, it can't be the training because she goes just as hard as you. I mean, we witness them training all the time when we are training and you both train hard."*

Maria conceded that I had a point there. I said to her, *"How's her [Racheal's] nutrition?"*

She answered, *"As far as I can tell, she doesn't eat that bad."*

I told Maria, *"Okay, give me a few days. I am going to talk to Johnny to see if he gave her a meal plan. And if he did, is she following it."*

Over the next few days, I saw Johnny and spoke to him about the conversation that I'd had with Maria. After getting a perspective on how things were, I told him, *"Fine, don't worry. You know I won't start training one of your clients because she wants to trainer hop. We don't do that."*

I proceeded to check up on the situation more thoroughly. Johnny assured me that he gave Racheal numerous meal plans. Was she following them? He didn't know. He also remembered her telling him that she had a physical done, and everything was fine.

As far as he could tell, he thought that maybe Racheal partied and drank a little too much on the weekends. I said to him, *"Yeah, but Maria also parties with her."* I explained, *"Don't get me wrong. I know that Racheal and Maria are two different people but if she has been training for over six months and has not lost a pound, don't you think something is wrong?"* I added, *"Have you asked her if she is stressed out?"*

He replied, *"No, but I'll tell you what. I am going to have this conversation with her in a cool, calm and collected way. Don't worry; I am going to get to the bottom of this and find out what's going on with her body."* I said, *"Sweet. Handle your business."*

Over the next few months, I witnessed Racheal training even harder than she did before. First thing came to my mind is that she and Johnny must have had a good conversation about the whole situation. This new performance of Racheal's during training made Maria step her game up too. She started training harder during every training session. Maria told me that she and Racheal haven't had a drink of alcohol in three months and that it started as just a friendly bet between the two of them.

Now you have two friends that are not drinking any alcohol, going by a strict meal plan supposedly and training extra hard.

Over this period, the only thing that changed was that Maria lost even more weight. Her body became so toned that it looked like it belonged on the cover of Shape magazine. One day a member made a joke to Racheal and Maria. He said, *"When both of you train, I believe all the results go straight to Maria."*

That comment was all it took. From that point on, Racheal and Maria started to feud. That particular remark upset Racheal a lot. She played it off by telling the member Frank that maybe he needed some new glasses. I started noticing that Racheal was not speaking to Maria that much before or after their training session. Then one day, I saw Racheal training at 7 pm on a Tuesday. I didn't think much of it until I saw her training at the exact same time on Tuesday again after that following Friday. Maria spilled the beans and told me, *"I think Racheal is upset at me or avoiding me. For what reason, I don't know. She told me last week that she's going to start training on different days from now on, but that was it."*

I said, *"Yeah, I saw her training on those days, and it surprised me. Because you two usually train at the same time."* I was a little taken aback. However, I didn't want to make it seem like I was instigating their feud or making matters any worse than they already were. So I said, *"Maybe it's a guy that she likes that comes on the same days and at the same time."*

Maria said, *"No, it's not that. We both have boyfriends."* I said, *"Maybe a new job schedule."* Maria answered, *"I don't know. All I know is that she's mad at me, and I don't know why."* Over the next few months, their friendship went downhill. It got to the point where neither one would speak to the other when they saw each other. One Monday, I decided to go on one of my usual runs. To my surprise, I saw Racheal at the park jogging, too. I don't know if it was the black yoga pants she was wearing, but it looked like she had lost 10lbs. We stopped and talked for about five minutes. I complimented her on her weight loss.

She thanked me and then immediately said, *"You are not going to believing this. I actually went to the doctor about a month ago and was diagnosed with hyperthyroidism. That's why it was so hard for me to lose any weight."*

I was puzzled, so I said to her, *"I thought you had a checkup before you started training?"*

She said, *"I might have told Johnny I did, but I hadn't because I thought it is just training, and that it's not that* serious. I could have saved myself a whole year of frustration and running around in a circle if I would've just taken the time and had a physical done."

I said, "Well, I am glad to see you found the answer to your problem."

"Me too," she said. "I'll see you at the gym on Monday most likely."

I said, "But I thought you stopped training on those days."

She said, "I did, but now I am back on my regular schedule."

Then she added, "I don't know if you noticed, but Maria and I weren't talking for a while. I called her the other day as a real friend should and apologized for my recent behavior. I explained to her how I wasn't feeling adequate since my body wasn't changing and hers was.

That I became jealous of her. I know I didn't do the right thing, but we all make mistakes. I then told her about my thyroid disorder. That I got it under control and I am now starting to lose weight. She said she was happy for me."

Racheal also admitted, "It wasn't my trainer's fault because I told him I had a physical done, and I hadn't."

So she and Maria had chitchatted, talked over their differences, and caught up. They both had agreed that it would be back to business at the gym on Monday, just like the old times. I told Racheal I was glad that she and Maria were friends again and that I would see her Monday.

Then I finished my run, thinking how Racheal could have avoided an entire year which went to waste and added to her stress if she would have just got a physical done! So that is pro tip#1: as soon as you plan to train, make sure you know what's up with your body. Get your physical done, and save yourself unnecessary trouble.

Chapter 2 – Remember Your Reason

Before you begin to train, ask yourself a few key questions.

Question 1: What is your reason for wanting to be more physically fit?

For some, training will involve wanting to do a 5K, getting a gym membership or CrossFit. Others might steer toward personal training. Whatever your reason is, stay focused and true to it. Everybody will have a reason. For example, some might have medical issues; some would want to be able to lift heavy weights; while others might want to sculpt their body to look better for their physical appearance. It is good to remind yourself of your reasons on a daily basis.

I often use an analogy that I share with any athletes I work with. I say to them, *"Look at your health as if it is a house."* Yes, this means considering the entire process of it. You lay the foundation of the house, and it is the strongest part of a house. It is the concert stab that the complete structure is built on. Without a strong foundation, your house will fall. So you have to look at your reason as if it is the strong concrete foundation for your house. Then, the goals that you set for yourself will be the wood that will be used to build that house. I repeat: don't focus on your goals so much that you forget your reason. This is because when you become too fixated on the goal, you will lose your motivation and inspiration but will remain dedicated to your goal that now has no purpose.

Once again, this will cause you to get lost. For example, imagine going to the gym five days a week. You do the same workout over and over again; you don't see any results but you constantly stick to the routine. This reminds me of what Einstein said about insanity: it is doing the same thing over and over, expecting a different result. You might think people don't do what I just mentioned, but the fact is that I see this a lot in some of the gyms that I frequent.

For example, there is this guy I know named Pat. I met him about three years ago when I was working out at this gym in Brooklyn. As I talked to him, I learned that he was a newbie at this gym stuff. He also told me that the only reason he had hit the gym was to lose weight so it can bring down his blood pressure. He said to me, *"I thought I would come to ask you for some advice. What exercises should I be doing to help me lose weight?"*

I told him, *"Today is your lucky day, Pat. I am a personal trainer."*

He said, *"No, I don't have any money for training."* Then he started to walk off. I called him back and said, *"Listen to me, Pat. I don't know you, and you don't know me, but if I give you a few routines to do, are you going to do them? Because if not, you are wasting your time and mine."*

He told me, *"I promise I will do them. Man, I need to bring down my blood pressure ASAP."*

I took his information on my phone over the next few days. I designed a training program and meal plan for him based on his predisposition, body type, goals, and his current age, height, and weight. I called Pat then told him I don't usually give out free information, but I know if I help you out, it will come back to me.

It's because I believe in the karmic law of 'what goes around comes around.' Pat then again promised me that he was going to follow the program. Pat said to email the plans I had created to him. Over the next few months, I would shoot Pat an email regularly just to see how everything was going.

Much to my surprise, Pat was following the plan; this is where some of the people who sign up for training really lack. Pat was making tremendous progress. Not only was his blood pressure going down but his body was starting to lean out. Pretty soon, I knew Pat would be back to his normal weight with a leaner and more sculpted physique than that before his blood pressure went up.

It was around a few months later that I passed Pat coming out of the gym as I was going in. I had to do a double take when I saw him. I stopped him and said, *"You're looking good, Pat."* He immediately thanked me again for helping him out, and said, *"I told you I would do the program."* He also told me that he looks and feels good, but most importantly, his blood pressure had finally started to go down.

Pat didn't know it, but right then and there, I felt the satisfaction at the success of the program I had designed for him. Just knowing I played a role in making Pat healthier was good enough for me. He then told me that when he gets some extra cash, he was going to send some my way. I smiled at his appreciation for my help.

As I was walking off, I told Pat to keep doing what he was doing and that in about four to five months he should be back to his normal self. I later found out that people had watched what Pat was doing. He had started to look better. Pat told everyone that he had started to exercise more. So a lot of people asked him if they could work out with him.

Soon, he started to let four guys that he made friends with at the gym work out with him. This was all fine and dandy at first. I am sure it felt good to Pat that he had four other guys to work out with. They would root each other on and spot each other on the heavy lifts they performed.

As time went on, however, Pat's new buddies started adding different exercises to the original program. Eventually, they had Pat doing fewer reps and sets than before. Now, the original program had been altered due to his new friends.

It was no longer the program that I had created after having considered Pat's history and condition. The next time I saw Pat, he was overweight again. He was standing in a circle with his buddies at the gym. They were getting all amped up for a bench press session. I said to Pat, *"What's up?"*

He said, *"What's going on?"* I told him I was about to do a little training. He shared with me that he had gotten stronger but had also put back on a lot of weight.

I said, *"Most likely your blood pressure is back sky high."*

He said, *"You are right."*

I guessed, *"You must have stopped doing the program."*

He agreed and said, *"I kinda stopped following the program about two months ago."* Then he added, *"Me and the boys sort of do whatever we are in the mood for that day."*

I told him, *"Well, all you have to do is just start back on the program and follow it."*

He told me, *"The boys said that the meal plan wasn't enough calories for me."*

"I see," I answered.

He thanked me once again then said, *"I am going to get back to the program one day, but for now it feels good working out with the boys."*

Now, I have quoted this example here to show you how your reason can become easily misplaced. You can become so far caught up in something that what matters the most can get pushed to the back of your mind instead of the front. We all like the feeling of belonging to something. Pat felt the same way, so he did not notice how his program was changing. Instead of what his body needed, his exercise routine was now based on his friends' feelings; his training was dependent on if his friends felt like doing an extra set or not. What happened was, Pat's new friends slowly influenced him to eat more carbs, not to mention empty ones.

By this, I mean those carbohydrates that have no nutritional value. Pat's meal plan and training program were quickly altered, and in a way that did not help his cause. Over the next year, I watched Pat let himself go. His belly and head became bigger and bigger. I witnessed Pat become fatter and fatter when only sometime back, he had achieved a leaner and healthier body.

Pat would say to me, *"The guys told him if I keep working out with them I'll be back to normal in no time."* Other than that, Pat started to avoid conversation with me. I could tell he felt he had let me down. Once again, I will remind you that working on your health is the same as building a house. Let your reason for wanting to be healthier be the strong concrete foundation for your house.

Make sure your reason is set in stone. Don't let others, friends or gym buddies or whoever, distance you from your reasons. As you can see in Pat's example, when you forget your reason, it becomes hard to stay on track. You are left running around in a circle. Pat started doing the same routine over and over with his buddies because it felt good to workout with the guys.

To me, that is an example of *"insanity."* So remember always your reason that is set in stone. Let it be the motivation and determination that you need. Use it to dedicate yourself to your goals. When you think about your reason on a daily basis and repeat it to yourself out loud, it is hard to steer you away from it.

Rule #1: Repeat your reason on a daily basis

Rule #2: Never forget rule 1.

Chapter 3 – Clarify Your Goals

After getting cleared by a doctor to participate in physical activity, the next step is to understand your reason. This means getting to know your goals. You have big goals and little ones. At the time that you start, make sure you are realistic with yourself. I say this because sometimes you can pick a goal so big that it just becomes too intimidating.

Then to top it off, you try to accomplish it in a timeframe that is practically impossible or even unhealthy. Getting into an exercise routine that is unhealthy for you will lead to unwanted stress; it comes from trying to execute a goal that was never set up in the proper order.

Remember this: set up equals execution. Without a good set up, it is hard to execute your plan. So pick realist goals from the start because when you don't, nine times out of ten you are setting yourself up for a recipe for disaster. As I mentioned before, I categorize all my goals into two categories: big and small ones. Then I break down each one into smaller categories.

For example day, week, monthly, and yearly goals are my DW & MY goals. My small goals category is broken down into what I call *DW* goals. The D stands for daily what can I do on a daily basis; these are the small goals that will help me accomplish my bigger goals. We do a lot of these daily goals in an automotive state which sometimes requires very little thinking, dedication or awareness. For this reason, they are usually taken for granted.

People should make it a goal to consume enough water on a daily basis. Yes, water makes up for about 60% of the average male body and 50% of the average female body. I have often seen people take drinking water for granted. I believe drinking water should not be one of the last things to worry about. In fact, if you ask me, it should be the first thing you keep track of on a daily basis.

Lack of water will cause you to become fatigued faster than you normally would. Staying hydrated during recovery will help your muscles receive the oxygen and nutrients it needs. Water also helps regulate your body temperature. Now without getting into full details about every function of the body that requires water, these are just a few I want to bring to your attention.

Since the focus is on exercise, if you know you are sweating it out doing your workout, then you need to put water back in your system. For example, before a workout you know you weighed a 150 pounds, and after your workout, you weigh a 148 pounds. That is a two-pound difference. Rule of thumb says drink 16 oz. of water for every pound of body weight lost during a workout.

So someone who loses two pounds should consume at least 32 oz. of water after their workout. With that being said, do you know how many times I have witnessed a client tap out during a training session due to dehydration or severe or muscle cramps? People know this fact, most of the times. Then why do they still overlook it so much?

I think the answer is a lot of people just forget drinking water with all the other little things they have to do throughout the day. For example, during their daily routine, they would not pause in whatever they are doing to tell themselves: *"Hey! Water up!"*

Now, when I talk of enough water consumption, I don't mean that you need to tote a jug of water around with you everywhere you go like some bodybuilders. What I am saying is, make it your business to know how much water you are consuming on a daily basis. This should be one of your small goals every day. Every time you consume some water make a note in your phone. At the end of the day, add it all up to see if you are consuming enough. If you are not, make the adjustments that should be made. Make this a daily goal, and hold yourself accountable for it. Another small daily goal that people overlook is rest. Rest, rest, rest. I can't say it enough!

Right now, as I speak do you know exactly how much rest you're getting every night? I've had so many people tell me, *"I just go to bed whenever I get tired."* Does this mean if you are tired at 5:00 p.m. on Monday, it's lights out? If you are tired at 11:00 p.m. on Tuesday, it's lights out and if you are tired at 3:00 a.m. on Wednesday, it's lights out? If you do something like this, then you have only succeeded in creating an awkward sleeping pattern - especially if you are someone who has to get up for work at 6:00 a.m. every morning.

A sleep pattern in which you do not get enough rest on a daily basis will definitely affect any type of workout. How do you expect to see any result at all from whatever type of exercise you do if you are not getting enough rest? Most people think results happen while they are in the gym. They think the more they work out, the more results they are going to see. I have seen people work out seven days a week, but when I talk to them, they tell me they are always tired. You don't say! Do you wonder why this happens? If you are in this state, it will definitely lead you to over-train. This, in turn, will cause you to feel fatigued all the time. You will also experience a loss of appetite; all of this will lead to restlessness. This is why it is so important to rest. The change doesn't happen in the gym. It happens when you rest. Resting is when your body rebuilds itself from all the strain and damage you have done to it.

Now get some rest and start repairing your body, and stop damaging it. Another one of my small goals which are part of my DW goals is TIME. So this makes water and rest a part of my daily goals and time as one of my weekly goals which make up my DW goals. How much time did you put into exercising this week? This is something you must keep track of on a weekly basis.

If you don't know how much you are exercising on a weekly basis, you will be all over the place. Imagine one week you exercise once on Monday, then the next week you exercise once on Friday, but the following week you exercise three times that week. Then the 4th week you don't exercise at all. If this is you, you shouldn't wonder why at the end of the month that you don't see any results!

It's as simple as this: you don't have an exercise schedule. For your workout to give you results, you must form and stick to a schedule. You don't have to train every day, but you should try your best to be consistent. If you exercise regularly, you have a greater chance of seeing the results you deserve. Now let's talk about the big goals which are my M-to-Y goals.

This stands for monthly and yearly goals. One example of my monthly goals is 'weigh in's.' I talked to so many clients who told me they don't want to get on a scale every day or once a week. A lot of them tell me it can become frustrating or depressing to see the digits. They would rather look at the bigger number at the end of the month. I guess it is more of a mental thing with them, and it seems to work.

I have witnessed clients that work harder doing a training session because they don't know how much weight they have already lost. On the other hand, if they know they only lost 1 lb. last week there are chances that they will become discouraged and only give a 50% effort during the training session. The next part of your M-to-Y goals is yearly. What would be a good, but realistic, yearly goal you could set for yourself for the year? Let's say you want to put on 10 pounds of lean muscle.

This would be an example of a yearly goal, except most people make it a monthly goal, then become extremely frustrated when things do not go their way. You do not want to lose your motivation, determination, because when this happens your dedication will go right out the window. This happens only because you didn't plan properly. You didn't set the right goals in the right time frame, and most of all you were not realistic with yourself.

Now, to stop this from happening, ask yourself: *is this goal really attainable in one year?* Adjust your answer according to the answer you reach. So think about the things that need to be done on a daily, weekly, and monthly basis – because they make up your big and small goals to complete that yearly goal. Then begin executing your plan, with the belief that you will get there.

Chapter 4 – Your Body Type

In my years of training, I have found one crucial fact: a lot of people go wrong with their body type. When they do not know their correct body type, naturally they do not align their exercises to suit their body type. When I ask people what body type are you, some answer 'I guess I'm tall' or 'I guess I'm fat.' It is clear that the average person thinks if they are not short then they must be tall, and if they are not skinny, then they must be fat.

This often leads them to select one of the four options that I just mentioned. When this happens, and it often does, I take it upon myself to explain to them the three different body types. They include ectomorph, endomorph, and mesomorph. Each body type is different in appearance. Also, each has its advantages and its disadvantages. A person can be more than one body type but still have one type predominantly.

When I tell people this, they are very surprised. It is like a moment of clarity just hit them. Then they immediately ask me, *"So what body type am I?"* So I point out the different traits of body types to them so they can identify theirs. Then I also explain some of the advantages and disadvantages of their body type. Some answer, *"You mean to tell me I can't be a bodybuilder?"* That's when I stop them and say: *"No, you can still be a bodybuilder. You are just going to have to work harder since you're an ectomorph."* Another one I get all the time is: *"I guess being a marathon runner is out of the question now since you told me I'm endomorph."* That's when I reassure them, *"You can still be a marathon runner. You are just going to have to work a little harder."*

One of my clients named Chris first walked up to me a few years ago, and said, *"I want to be able to do a marathon."* I know that he would be able to be a marathon runner because of his ectomorph physique. Don't get me wrong, he would still have to work hard, but he would be doing something that his body was basically bred for. So I knew in due time he would complete his first marathon. And as of now, he's killing it. He does the marathon every year.

I have not revealed this information to you to discourage you in any way. I give you this information so you can understand what type of exercise, training or sport you will most likely be good at, keeping in mind your body type. Instead of you jumping headfirst into any type of exercise or training, you should know your body type. Without doing your research, your chances of being successful at it are slim.

Now, let's look at the three graphs I have designed for you on body types and their traits. I would like you to take the time and pick out the body type that best fits you.

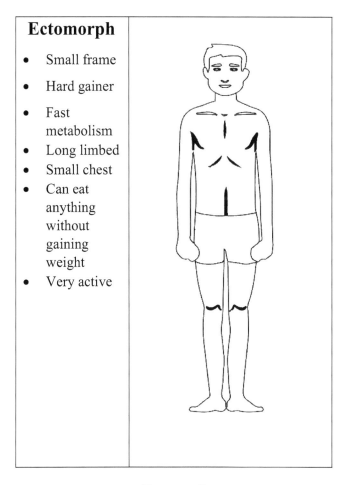

Ectomorph

- Small frame
- Hard gainer
- Fast metabolism
- Long limbed
- Small chest
- Can eat anything without gaining weight
- Very active

Ectomorph

Mesomorph

- Athletic
- Absolutely strong
- Broad shoulders
- Put on muscle easily
- Well defined muscles
- Muscular chest
- Wide clavicles

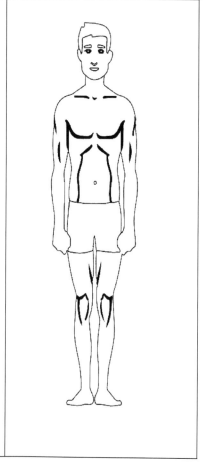

Endomorph

- Stocky
- Barely any muscle definition
- Round body
- Short limbs
- Lose weight slowly
- Gain muscle and fat easily
- Thick arms and legs

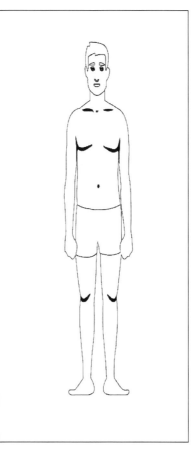

Some of you probably had no problem picking out your body type. As soon as you read it, you told yourself: that's me, 110%! Some of you probably had a little problem, and you felt that you had a couple of traits of a different type, apart from the main type that you selected. Don't be confused by this. It happens a lot. It is normal for a person to be more than one body type. A person can be little mesomorph, a lot of ectomorph, but at the end of the day, they would still be an Ectomorph because that is their predominant type.

It is the body type they have the most traits of. Now since you know this, how will you use this information to help you? Can you see yourself selecting a different sport, exercise or training to put yourself into, keeping in mind your body type? If your sport, training or exercise stays the same, will you change your method of approach now that you know this?

Another question to ask yourself is: does this newfound knowledge affect your eating? Ask yourself: *"Since I have this new insight, should my nutrition change?"* Now that you know some of the advantages and disadvantages of your body type, you should be able to tweak the physical activity of your choice to your advantage!

Chapter 5 – Tailor Your Training around Your Body Type

Training is not a one size fits all activity. Many people seem to be unaware of the fact, though. For training to be effective and for you to meet your goals, you have to tailor your training around your body type. Now ask yourself: *how can I go about doing this?*

Setting Goals

The first step is to figure out your goals. What is it that you want to accomplish? Are you someone who wants to lose weight? Are you trying to gain weight? Or is your goal to get stronger legs? Whatever the case may be, you have to realize that your goals will eventually change as you proceed. When this happens, your training will change too.

Now, you may be the kind of a person who doesn't like to set that many goals right at the start. You may fear being overwhelmed by thinking of all the changes when you have only begun. Well, you should know that your training will still have to change for your body to maintain what it has at present.

You might think, *"But why can't I do what I have been doing for some time now?"* The answer is that doing the same thing over and over again will, after a time, stop giving you results. It would not produce the same effect on your body as it once did when you first started with it.

My Body Type + Goals = Physical Activity

For example, if you have been lifting weights, after a while you will need to adjust the weight and rep ranges. It is because your body can stand a little bit more now. You need to give your body more to even produce the same results as before. It is all about the science of your body.

Adapt and Change

The one fact about our bodies when it comes to training is this: bodies adapt quickly. Think of it like this. You set a goal for yourself. You started lifting weights, but after some time, your body adapted to the training. Now, if you keep doing the same training you were doing before, your body will hardly change. So what you need to do is to change the training. Modify your training routine to keep getting the results you want.

To help you better understand this, I have set up a few tables on the next page. What you have to do now is go to the three tables that I have created according to body type. Look at the figures and identify your body type. Then read the graph to give yourself a better understanding of where you should start with your training and where you should take it next.

Worksheet Instructions

- Look at all the tables and find which one is your body type.

- Once you have selected your body type, proceed to the column for goals and write down one of your goals. Don't worry if you have more than one goal. You can list them as shown from the first goal to the second goal and so on.

- After you have filled in your body type and your goals, the last thing is to select the type of physical activity that will accommodate your body to help you meet your goals. This is what we talked about in the previous pages as well.

Table 1: Ectomorph Body Type

Body type	Goals	Physical Activity
Ectomorph Person	First: I want to get bigger	<ul><li>Gym</li><li>Lifting weight</li><li>Heavy weights</li><li>3 to 5 rep range</li></ul>
	Second:	
	Third:	
	Fourth:	

Table 2: Endomorph Body Type

Body type	Goals	Physical Activity
Endomorph Person	First: I want to lose weight	• HIIT training
	Second:	
	Third:	
	Fourth:	

Table 3: Mesomorph Body Type

Body type	Goals	Physical Activity
Mesomorph Person	First: I want to rip up.	• 2 to 3 cardio sessions • A week with weight training (moderate to heavy weights) • 12 to 12 rep range, 4 days a week
	Second:	
	Third:	
	Fourth:	

The Next Step

For some of you, this is going to be easy. Then, there would be some of you who will make this more complicated than it is. I am here to tell you: **It's OK!** This is just a formula that I go by. I don't want you to feel like you are failing a test. If this is helpful to you, please use it and repeat it with whatever physical activity you choose to participate in.

As more time will pass, you will notice that as your goals change, your physical activity will change too. For example, a person who was going to the gym to lose weight now wants to put on a little muscle. So he might stop doing so much cardio, and insert two days of resistance training to the program.

Then in other cases, your physical activity might switch from you being in the gym to an entirely different setting and atmosphere – like running outside. Yes, you might be someone that needs to run outside in a certain temperature and at a certain elevated height to train your respiratory system. For example, people who participate in altitude training compete or train at normal sea level.

Now, you need to keep track of your physical activity over a period of time. Is it changing at all? If it isn't changing, then it is a definite sign that you need to set more goals. Don't get discouraged by this. Rather, you should welcome it with open arms. Start thinking of goals as new challenges! Like they say, if it doesn't challenge you it won't change you!

Chapter 6 – Safety

Safety is the least talked about aspect of training. The athletes I train will tell you how big I am on safety. So it makes sense that I would dedicate an entire chapter to safety while training. They will also tell you that one of my mains slogans that they hear me say all the time: *hard-headed people are always injured.* And I mean this mentally and physically, however, you want to look at it.

Don't get me wrong – I am not saying that injury is entirely avoidable during training. People will have some injuries here and there when they train. The injuries may occur due to people challenging themselves or making simple mistakes like dropping a weight on their foot. However, most of the injuries that I have seen over a period of time as a personal trainer happened because people did not listen.

Every gym has those five or ten members who are always bandaged up. One month it is a knee brace, the next month it is an ankle brace, followed by an elbow brace. The only thing missing is a neck brace for a full body cast. I am not saying any of this to be funny. I am just pointing out facts. You would think after all these injuries – sustaining them or seeing other sustain them – people would start training safely. I know I would if I were in their place. But the sad truth is that people hate to take precautions. Suppose you have a guy named Tom who wants to strengthen his legs. However, Tom has a weak lower back from injuries that he sustained previously.

Considering the condition of his body, it would be safe to say that Tom shouldn't be doing deadlifts. If this is the case, you take the barbell deadlifts out of your program and use the trap bar which is much safer for you. This is what safety in the gym is about – developing a program that suits the needs of your body and doesn't push you to the extent that you end up being injured.

Another thing that I notice is that a lot of people like to bench press without a spot. I don't know why they do that. It only takes five seconds to ask someone to spot you, and it takes five months for you to recover from an injury. Another thing I witness is a lot of ego lifting. I am pretty sure every person in America who goes to the gym has seen this; this is precisely what later leads to injury.

If you train regularly, you need to ask yourself: *"When I leave the gym from exercising am I in pain for the next few days?"* When I say pain, I am not talking about Delayed Onset

Muscle Soreness (DOMS). I am talking about bodily pain to where you feel as if you are injured. Since it is your body, you should know how long this has been going on. The reason I asked you to assess any physical pain you might experience is because the body's little aches and pains are telltale signs that something is wrong.

This usually happens before an injury. I am just using this as an example, so I don't have to go into every exercise and talk about the safest way to do them. Most people do not know there is a certain way an exercise should be done. For example, when it comes to lifting weight, a beginner usually thinks if he or she can move the weight from Point A to Point B, they are doing it right.

They never actually realize that for every exercise there is a specific way you should adjust your body to prevent injury, that there is a correct way to perform any exercise. This is called 'correct form.' It doesn't matter if you are lifting 300 lbs. or doing one pushup. You should always use correct form, and perform them the right way.

Don't get me wrong; I know you are going to have those days where you are crunched for time which will lead you to speed through your workout. When this happens, you must still pay attention to your form because usually the faster you speed through any exercise, the more you start to lose form. And once again, when the form is gone injury can occur.

To top it off, since muscle has memory, when you perform the same exercise again any time in the future, you will go at the same speed even when you are not in a rush. This increases the chances of injury even more. I repeat: any exercise you do has a correct way in which it should be performed. It doesn't matter if you are lifting weight, running, or using dip bars in the park. Every exercise has a correct way it should be performed to lessen your chance of injury.

It is a fact that when your form is right, your strength will increase faster. Then you won't have to do the ego lift, which I will talk about in detail later. First, let me show you an example of the three exercises I see performed all the time with bad form.

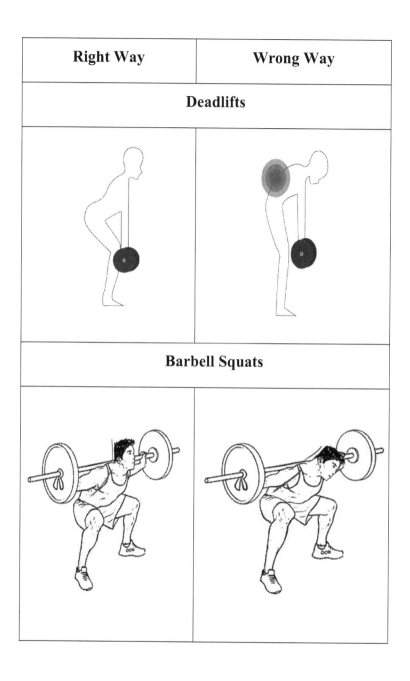

Right Way	Wrong Way
Deadlifts	
Barbell Squats	

Shoulder Press

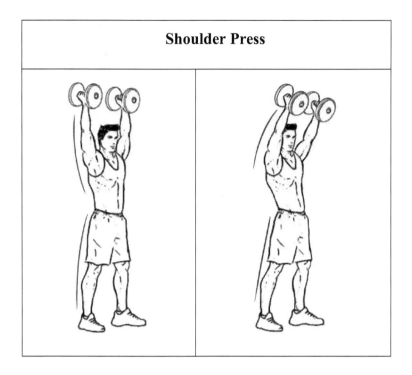

The Ego Lift

The ego lift is another fast way to get injured. If you don't know what I'm talking about ego lift is when you see someone add more weight than they can handle to an exercise and try to perform it. Instead of taking some of the weight off, he or she will continue to try to lift the weight, which is too heavy, with improper form. As we speak, I guarantee you that there is someone in your gym doing this right now.

A lot of people do this because they want to give others the impression that they can lift a lot of weight. So yes, this is a real ego thing. Instead of using correct form to get stronger so that eventually they will be able to lift the weight, they would rather use improper form and pretend to be strong enough to lift weight when they are not. As this goes on, a person who ego lifts will eventually do it with every type of lift they do. This, once again, increases their chance of getting an injury.

It is obvious that a person who does this has no clue about what is going on. It is as if the thought never occurred to them to lower the weight on whatever lift they are doing and lift the weight with correct form. If they do this, then in time they will be able to go back to that same heavy weight as before, and eventually lift it the right way because they would have gotten stronger.

I know me speaking on form probably doesn't come off as a big surprise to you – after all, I *am* a trainer, and I care about form for a living – but think back to your time in the gym. I am pretty sure if any of you have been injured in the gym before it was because your form was not correct. This is why it is important to have correct form. Now, if you haven't been injured before, do not think of yourself as an exception.

We have all been guilty of doing exercise the wrong way at one point or another. However, the only way to get better at something is to learn and practice, and the only way to do that is to put the ego aside. Don't be afraid to ask the trainer at your gym the correct form. Also, you can take some time out to watch credible videos on specific exercises you are trying to perform. Either way, when you expand your knowledge on the subject, you will most likely learn the right way to do it. It is safe to say that the less you know about an exercise, the greater your chances are at performing it wrong.

This could lead to an injury. Now I want you to think when you are in the gym, performing different types of exercises, are you doing them in the safest way possible? How many of you notice that there are eight or ten exercises you do that could lead to a quick injury, just because you are trying to hit a certain muscle group? When you think about it, there are probably three or more different exercise for each of those eight that will hit the same muscle group with a lesser chance of injury. As we conclude chapter 6, I say it again: safety, safety, safety! Pay attention to your surroundings when you're exercising. Put the ego lift to the side. Last but not least, try your best to use the correct form!

Chapter 7 – Nutrition

A lot of people don't realize the importance of nutrition. Many people wake up and eat whatever they want every day, never taking the time to calculate how many calories they are consuming on a daily basis. It is a known fact that you are what you eat. If you eat unhealthy food, then you are going to feel unhealthy. I challenge you to start making healthier food choices. First, take the time out and find out what food allergies you have, if you don't know them already.

Next, I want you to start keeping track of everything you eat for 24 hours on your phone. Repeat the same for three more days. Once you have gathered your data, I want you to see how much of a difference is there in your diet in the three days. One day you might have consumed 1200 calories, other days you probably consumed 2200. I want you to know this fact: you want your calories to be consistent as much as possible on a daily basis.

Now, instead of playing the guessing game, which a lot of people do, you need to figure out how many calories you should be consuming on a daily basis. To do this, you need to figure out your RMR, which is your resting metabolic rate. If you were to sit for 24 hours without doing anything at all, your body would still burn a certain amount of energy. This amount of energy that is burned is the least amount of calories you need to consume on a daily basis. When you are doing any physical activity, and you are not consuming enough calories, then you will feel tired and fatigued.

So always make sure you consume a certain amount of calories – that is the same amount or more than your RMR, and not below it. Once you establish your caloric intake, your goal is to try to hit that number every day. You can do this by dividing meals. You can track the calorie content of everything you eat. For some people tracking every little thing they eat is frustrating; then there are also some people who have no problem doing this. Now, once you start consuming your target amount of calories that you set out for on a regular basis, it is your job to start taking notes.

Start taking notes in your phone. Ask yourself questions regularly such as: Did I lose any weight this week? Has my energy level been consistent? As you start to keep track of your nutrition intake and strive to maintain consistency in it, you will soon begin to notice a pattern about the way that you feel. All of this stems from the pattern of eating that you establish. Now your next step will be one of the biggest steps in your nutrition plan.

I like adding this step last because most people get overwhelmed when you start talking about switching out everything they eat for new food. I want you to make sure everything on your calorie list is a healthy food choice. Yes, I know this isn't easy, so I would like you to take it one meal at a time. This allows you to wing yourself off the bad food that is empty calories.

It is kind of like a person smoking cigarettes; he or she cannot quit overnight. Similarly, I don't expect you to overhaul your diet overnight. People don't start eating unhealthy food overnight, and they can't stop eating the same food in a matter of days. So take it meal by meal to wing yourself off the bad food. As you modify your diet, create some structure at the same time. I say this because we are creatures of habit. If you develop a pattern and stick to the routine, you will start following it automatically every day. Now, you may ask: what is healthy food? Well, healthy food means a combination of things: it means eating a variety of foods that maintain your health, make you feel good, and give you energy. Below, we have the Food Pyramid to help you distinguish between healthy and unhealthy food.

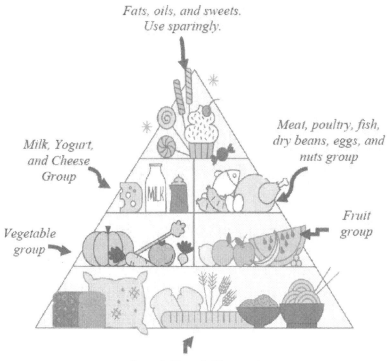

Fats, oils, and sweets.
Use sparingly.

Meat, poultry, fish,
dry beans, eggs, and
nuts group

Milk, Yogurt,
and Cheese
Group

Fruit
group

Vegetable
group

Bread, Cereal, Rice and
Pasta Group

Now, if you have been following me, your total daily calories should consist of a certain amount of carbs, proteins, fats, water, vitamins, and minerals. You will get your energy from carbs, proteins, and fats. Let's take this one step at a time. We will start with carbs. Carbs are short for carbohydrates; they are any large group of organic compounds occurring in food and living tissues and including sugars starch and cellulose. They contain hydrogen and oxygen in the same ratio as water and typically can be broken down to release energy in the animal body. This is the dictionary's definition, which might get confusing. So to put it in layman terms, carbohydrates are energy.

I want you to look at the daily calorie list that you made on your phone and determine how much of it is carbs and how much are proteins, and fats. Once you add up the number of carbs, you will need to multiply it by 4, because one gram of carbs contains four calories. Whatever number you get you will need to figure out what percentage of your total calories is this number. This can be done by using a calculator. For example:

- Let's say you consume 2500 calories on a daily basis
- You add up 300 in carbs, then multiply it by 4; this equal 1200.
- You would then need to express 1200 in terms of percentage of 2500 – which is 48%.

After you find your percentage for your carbohydrates, you can use the same formula you just did for finding your percentage of protein consumed on a daily basis, because every gram of protein also has four calories. When it comes to fat, you can use the same formula as you did for your carbs and protein, but instead of multiplying by four you will be multiplying it by nine because fat has nine calories for each gram.

As you now take a look at the three numbers you have and what percentages they equal, are you satisfied with it? Did you realize you were consuming this percentage of fats, carbs, and proteins? Or did you think it was a little more or less of each? Whatever the case may be, now you can calculate your caloric intake. Use the exact formula as you did before, then adjust the figures as you need to, either lowering or adding each of the three – carb, protein, and fat – that you see fit for your needs.

We also must talk about the importance of vitamins and minerals. You should take your vitamins on a daily basis. For all of you wondering about the difference between two – well, vitamins are organic, and minerals are inorganic. They both perform hundreds of roles in the body, from converting food into energy to repairing cell damage, which anybody exercising should be concerned about.

Make sure you do not consume an excess amount of vitamins and minerals. Now, last but not least, as we talk about nutrition, we must talk about complex carbohydrates and simple carbohydrates. Simple carbohydrates are broken down by the body quickly, and they raise your insulin level.

Whenever your insulin level rises, it gives your body the opportunity to store fat. Complex carbohydrates take longer to digest, and are broken down by the body slowly.

They do not raise the insulin level as rapidly, so your body stays in a metabolic state, also called the fat burning state. Now, look at your daily caloric intake list and convert as many simple carbohydrates as you can into complex carbohydrates, especially if your goal is weight loss. Your meal plan is starting to come together. As you implement all these adjustments into your daily eating habits, you will start to feel healthier, leaner, and more energetic.

The question I get most after all these new feelings acquired is: *when should I work out?* You should eat 90 minutes before your workout. Therefore, if you are working out at 12:00 pm., the last amount of food you should have consumed should have been at 10:30 and no later than that. This gives your body time to digest the food. If not, your body will have to work twice as hard to digest your food. So remember this fact: scheduling your workout around your mealtime makes a significant difference!

Chapter 8 – Consistency

This chapter is all about consistency. How consistent are you with your training and nutrition? This is a very important question because I am a firm believer that the way you do one thing, is the way you do everything. So ask yourself, are you the type of a person that falls off track every two weeks or are you the type of a person that makes a plan and sticks to it? If you belong to the second category, then it is all good. However, if you belong to the first type that I mentioned here, then we must talk about it.

Back in Chapter 2, we talked about remembering your reason. What was your reason? Whatever your reason is, it has to be something that motivates you. This is the only way you will stay focused on your fitness journey. A lot of people pick reasons that do not motivate them at all. This isn't a small matter; when something doesn't motivate you, then it doesn't stimulate the brain which makes it ten times harder to keep going. You need to keep your reason at the forefront of your mind to create any type of consistency in your training routine.

I know this can be very hard for some of you but stop one second and think about every other hard situation that you made it through when you thought you couldn't. The only difference is your training is voluntary; since you have the choice to train consistently or not, some of you will just choose not to be consistent. Stop thinking of the word choice as 'I can' or 'I cannot.'

I say that because choice means an act; it is a clear indicator that means you do something whether or not it is big. Instead of thinking *"I don't have to do anything at all"* think differently. To retrain your brain, you must create a new thought process so you will stop reverting to old negative habits of failure.

It is a known fact that when you think about things that make you happy throughout the day, it will keep your mind stimulated. A lot of you look at your training and nutrition as if it is something you hate doing or a job that is hard or just something to get over with. As you use negative words, you put yourself in a state of mind which does not help you develop consistency.

When you have a negative thought process, it is because you think of something as something bad. This makes it so much harder for you to stay on track. You will not remain motivated to exercise because the idea of training, with its negative associations, will not be on your mind through the day. Ask yourself the question: *"When was the last time I constantly thought of things I don't like doing?"* Usually, things we don't like doing like – such as things that take time and hard work – we put them at the back of our minds.

As we do that, we cannot possibly achieve them as we are never thinking about them. The solution is to change our thought process. From now on, think of your consistency with training and nutrition as a win-win situation. I want you to realize there's no feeling involved in this because it is you who are administering the test. There is no reason for you to associate your consistency with the word 'bad' or 'fail'; instead, think of the word 'passing' constantly. Yes, I said 'passing.' Throughout the day, tell yourself you are passing because passing is a process that is not finished yet.

The only differentiation you make when you think of passing is: do you want to pass now or later? Either way, you're passing. There is no good or bad or wrong answer. As you begin to think this way, it would change your thought process. Yes, I apply the word consistency to your training and nutrition because to be consistent is a habit. Some of us take longer than others to develop this habit, but that's all right because there is no timeframe on it.

This means if you really put your mind to it you can start developing that habit right now. The only way to do that is to hold yourself accountable to your training and nutrition is by being consistent. Now as we go deeper into your thought process, I want you to ask yourself this question: *"Why am I not consistent?"* Take a few minutes out and let it marinate. Also, please be honest with yourself; if you aren't, you are only fooling yourself.

Remember, the way you do one thing is the way you do everything. Now, whatever your answer is, I am here to tell you that that's not the real answer. Whatever you just wrote down or came up with in your mind is just an excuse for the real question at hand. The real answer at the end of the day, no matter how you look at it, is that you haven't made being consistent a priority.

When you make it a priority to be consistent with your training and nutrition, not only will this become a habit but you will start to develop your craft. So make it a priority to be consistent. Some of you will ask: *How do I do this?* Take one second and think. You make it a priority to do everything else in your life that matters right! Then you need to start telling yourself that you are training and your nutrition is a priority.

Tell yourself that nutrition matters so you can develop the habit of being consistent. One problem is a lot of you can't see the result yet of how you want your bodies to look or feel. It is hard to make something matter to you that you can't see. That's why I revert to one of my keywords: 'passing.' Just tell yourself you are passing and enjoy the ride. Another way to become consistent is to make your training and nutrition fun.

What I mean by consistency is training and consuming a certain amount of calories a day. That doesn't mean you can't switch up your training to make it fun or more interesting. The same applies to your nutrition. It doesn't have to be the same old dull food all the time. You can go for different food options that taste delicious to you as long as the criteria of nutrients and calories are met.

Switching things to keep them interesting will make you want to do it more. As time goes on, you will start to be consistent. It will come as effortlessly to you as, for example, putting on your shoes does every morning. You wake up, put your shoes on, and get it over with. We do this in an automatic state. This is how I would like you to start doing your training and nutrition. Remember, there is no timeframe on when you will master the habit of consistency, both mental and physical, but when it does, it will start to bring you several steps closer to your goals.

Chapter 9 – Recovery

In Chapter 9, we are going to talk about the last key factor of your training. Now, this is the aspect that is a must-do if you wish to see the results you want. For some reasons, this last key factor is taken for granted all the time. I cannot stress the importance of it enough when it comes to training yielding the results you want. I am talking about recovery, ladies, and gentlemen.

How much recovery do you need in between workouts? Well, that would all depend on the intensity level of that workout. Let's say you train for an hour and your intensity level was pretty high. If that is the case, then I would recommend waiting 48 hours at least until working out again at that same muscle group at the same intensity.

Now, don't get this hour of work confused with an hour of chatting. The reason why I bring that up is because I see it all the time. I watch people come to the gym for one hour, out of which they spend 40 minutes talking; and to top it off, they do this five days a week. Once you do the math at the end of the week, you can see that they only worked out for a total of 1 hour and 40 minutes, because they were chatting about protein, who's hot and who's not. This is a certain recipe for disaster because when the weekend rolls around the same person will say Saturday and Sunday are my rest days. Yep, this routine never fails. So if this is you, let's break down the facts: you are working out less than two hours a week, and the intensity level isn't high at all, because you are constantly talking and are probably not focused.

It would be safe to say that you shouldn't be concerned with recovery at all because you haven't done any level of damage to your body, big or small. I see this happen all the time. So when a person like this ask me about recovery, I immediately say to them, *"Why are you worried about recovery?"* The answer that I get is the same all the time: *"Because I don't want to over-train."*

This is the time that I have to tell them the truth: *"You don't have to worry about overtraining, because you don't train hard enough."* I don't leave things off at that point but proceed to break down the numbers so they can see the truth: they work out for less than 2 hours a week, just like I calculated because of all the talking. I don't do this to be rude. I just state the facts, so maybe they will change the situation.

Now for those of you that have worked out hard enough – you definitely need these recovery days. Some people like taking one day on one day off; or they would take two days on one day off. Also, don't forget about the famous four-day split. The good thing is that depending on your intensity level; you can try out any of the three to see which one works best for you. Regardless of which one you pick, you will still want to switch around these recovery days to incorporate some change in your pattern.

Let's talk about what you will be doing on these recovery days. Before you take off recovery days, you would first have to decide this: are you going to do active recovery or passive recovery? Some of you are probably wondering: what's the difference? Well, passive recovery is letting the body completely rest from exercise, and active recovery is any low-intensity exercise. So if you are someone who goes for passive recovery then on your off days, you wouldn't be working out at all. You should be home watching Netflix.

For those of you doing active recovery, you have some options to choose from.

- You can do a light workout that mimics the movements from the day before if you like; this will help recovery because it will send an adequate amount of blood flow to the muscles and this helps circulation to transport nutrients for repair.

- You can choose to do yoga as long as it is not intense; this will also help you with Delayed Onset Muscle Soreness (DOMS) by lengthening the muscles and tendons.
- You could also choose to get a massage if you like. This always helps loosens your muscles and reduces the tightness.
- You can do the infrared sauna which increases blood flow and can reduce pain.
- You can do cryotherapy which also reduces inflammation.

Now, these are just a handful of options; there are a lot more for you to choose from. I recommend you try out a few to see which one your body agrees with best. Also, depending on the level of your workout you might switch it up each time. One week you might do cryotherapy, the next week you might want to do yoga, and a week after that you might get a massage. Play around with your recovery activities to recover from the amount of damage that was done to your body.

Some of you, however, just can't do this. You don't give your body time to recover as you are an active person by nature and just have to be doing something. So you do not rest. Even when you know you are supposed to be doing active recovery, you tend to turn that recovery session into a full intense workout, because you are just hardheaded.

I am here to tell you that not taking time to recover will kill your results every single time. It is necessary for you to become disciplined, and tone it down at certain times. By doing this, you are basically nursing your body. You are giving your body the time that it needs to repair. If you do this, I promise your results will be far greater than what they are now.

Now I want you to go over this chapter, and make a recovery schedule based on your current training plan. I am pretty sure your training varies so your recovery should vary, too. Do not be afraid to try one of these techniques that you haven't tried before. Now, as you do any form of recovery, remember not to take it for granted and do exactly what you are supposed to: *recover!*

Chapter 10 – Track Your Results

Now after you have covered everything that I talked of in the previous chapters, I think it is appropriate to base the last chapter of the book on tracking your results. Until you have tracked the results of your training, you will not understand the importance of it. So many people go to the gym, and just aimlessly do things, meaning that they have no routine or no idea what they would like to do. They jump from machine to machine, just to get a switch or to mimic what they see others do. But the reality of it is that they are both bad ideas.

For one, if you are someone who works a job where you sit at a desk all day, the last thing you want to do when you come to the gym is only to use machines where you are sitting; this defeats the purpose of your workout, plus it's lazy. Let's get you up moving around and get those hips open. Sitting for eight hours at work then coming to the gym and sitting, even more, is not good at all.

You are not stretching your hip flexors to lengthen the muscles from sitting all day so your hip flexors will remain short; this will cause those tight hips only to get worse if you don't address the issue. Now, just because you see someone do an exercise or you pull a routine off on Instagram doesn't mean that that particular routine is for you.

When I tell a person this, the first thing they tell me is something like this: *"She and I look the same. We are both 5'2 and love doing glute workouts."* I say to them, *"Yeah, but you don't move the same. How about we design a program specifically for you to fix your imbalances so you can move better? Then eventually you will be able to do the movements you're trying to mimic while working on your glutes at the same time."*

I give this example so you can see why you should track your results because for you to track your results, you must track what you are doing. The only way to do that is to have a routine specifically designed to improve your physical capabilities. It is just like the saying goes: you have to know where you come from to know where you're going. It is the same with training programs. Let's see where you are at right now; then we can project where you could go.

Now, when you track your results, you will be able to tell how much progress you have made in many areas. There are many ways to do this. I say this because you might just be that person who hops on a scale, and on not finding it move the way you want, you start to think that you are not making any progress. So before you get discouraged, you should do a skin fold test.

I say this just because the scale didn't move doesn't mean you have not lost any inches. This is a prime example of your body converting to more lean body weight. Has your flexibility improved? You can find that out if you can touch your toes now when you couldn't touch them before. Or has your stamina improved? Over the past months of your training, these are some of the things you should keep track of.

If you can do more work in an hour than you could before then yes, your stamina has improved. You probably started doing box jumps on the low box, and now you are doing them on the high box; this means your vertical jump has improved. These are some of the ways to track your progress, but many people don't keep track. You can say that if you don't keep track, you are taking your training for granted.

This is because as soon as you get discouraged, you don't have any proof to verify your results. And when you don't have any proof of something, it is a little bit like it never happened.

So please track your results in the future. Trust me it will help you more than it will hinder you or take up your time. This is the key to your entire training program.

What do you think you are training for? Depending on the outcome of your results, you will know if you need to tweak your training program to be able to accomplish whatever goal you set for yourself. Now when you don't track your results, it is like you are shooting in the dark. I don't know about you, but I would like to see my target, and the only way to do this is to track your progress so you know where you are at and where you would like to go.

As I leave you with that thought, I ask you to aim and shoot. Because like they say, the body only achieves what the mind believes.

Until next time, my friends.

Made in the USA
Middletown, DE
15 February 2019